THE POCKET BOOK OF

Sex&Chocolate

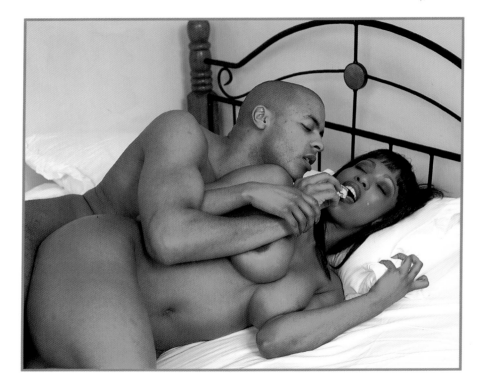

THE POCKET BOOK OF

Sex & Chocolate

What more could a body want?

Richard Craze

Hunter House
PUBLISHERS

For further information, please contact:
Hunter House Inc., Publishers
P.O. Box 2914, Alameda CA 94501-0914

Designed for Godsfield Press by
The Bridgewater Book Company

Studio photography by Peter Pugh-Cook
The publishers would like to thank the following for the use of pictures:
Corbis p. 11, p. 12 and p. 38

Library of Congress CIP data is available

ISBN 0-89793-320-6 (pb)

Printed in Hong Kong

ORDERING INFORMATION
Trade bookstores and wholesalers in the U.S. and Canada, please contact Publishers Group West
Tel: 1-800-788-3213 Fax: (510) 528 3444

Hunter House books are available for bulk sales at discounts to qualifying community and health-care organizations.
For details, please contact:
Special Sales Department
Hunter House Inc., P.O. Box 2914, Alameda CA 94501-0914

Tel: (510) 865 5282 Fax: (510) 865 4295
e-mail: ordering@hunterhouse.com

Individuals can order our books from most bookstores, or by calling 1-800-266-5592
or at **www.hunterhouse.com**

9 8 7 6 5 4 3 2 1 First Edition 01 02 03 04 05

CONTENTS

INTRODUCTION

What is it about chocolate that is so sensual, so satisfying,
so delicious, and so very sexy? And what is it about sex that is so sensual,
so satisfying, so delicious, and so very chocolatey?

Sex and chocolate are the nearest we'll get to heaven while still alive. Both of them lift our mood, calm our restless passions, lift our spirits and make us happy, and generally enhance our well-being. Without them we are lesser beings. And just imagine combining the two of them—what new and delicious heights of lust and gratification could we aspire to and reach?

DON'T EAT MORE, EAT BETTER
There is a whole lot of stuff about sex that keeps all of us restrained by convention. Sometimes it is seen as taboo, something that you shouldn't be indulging in. The same goes for chocolate. We fear being seen eating too much. We worry about putting on weight. And, worst of all, we view chocolate as somehow sinful or shameful.

Well, this is the book you've been waiting for. The book of sex and chocolate. Now you can indulge yourself—go on, wallow in all your delightful sinfulness. Life's too short to deny yourself anything.

RIGHT *You can share chocolate with whoever you like—your best friend or your lover—as long as you enjoy it.*

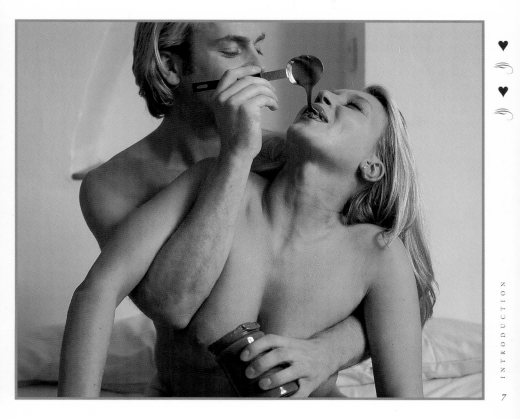

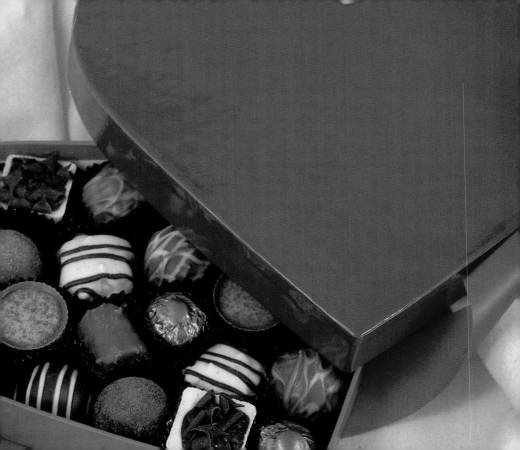

A HISTORY OF
CHOCOLATE

*From the very first time chocolate was "discovered" in the
New World it has been associated with sex. And quite rightly so. It
certainly seems to have many properties that might, understandably,
make some people consider it to be an aphrodisiac. It was Columbus
himself who first brought chocolate back to the Old World in 1502,
despite finding the drink unpalatable and bitter.
Seventeen years later, Cortés arrived at the Aztec capital of
Tenochtitlan, where he was received by the Emperor Montezuma.
And it was there that the legendary properties of chocolate were first
discovered. But we jump ahead of ourselves. The real history of
chocolate starts long before the Aztecs themselves.*

THE TREE

Three thousand years ago in an area south of Veracruz on the Gulf of Mexico, the earliest Mesoamerican civilization began. The people of this civilization were the Olmecs. They cultivated a tree that bore fruits known as cacao.

The Olmecs were replaced by the Mayans around the fourth century AD, and they named the tree that bore these fruits *cacahuaquchtl*, which just means "the tree." They considered no other tree worthy of bearing a name. When you had this tree, what use was any other? The Olmecs believed the seed pods were an offering from the gods, and were the first real chocolate drinkers. Some Mayan hieroglyphs that have survived show chocolate being thickened with maize meal and flavored with chilies, but it was always poured from a great height to produce the essential froth.

I'LL BE BACK

After the Mayans came the Toltecs, who worshiped the great god Quetzalcoatl. This god's role was to bring the seeds of the cacao tree from Paradise to earth for the benefit of all humankind. Quetzalcoatl, according to legend, left the area after going insane but promised to return on a specific date. This story is important as it might explain why the Spaniards were able to penetrate so far into Aztec country.

RIGHT *The mighty cacao tree growing in the wild, showing the huge pods that make it so famous.*

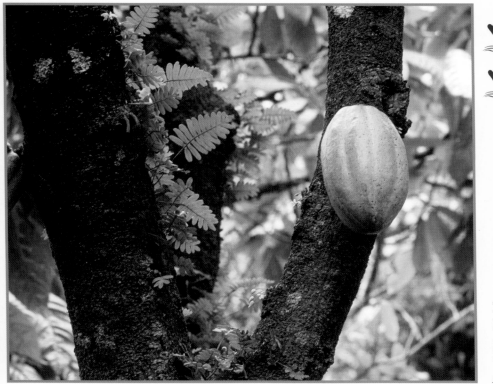

After the Toltecs, the area was settled by the Aztecs. They inherited much of the Toltec religion including waiting for the return of Quetzalcoatl. They also inherited the cacao tree and learned the pleasures that drinking chocolate could bring.

1519

Guess what happened in 1519? Yep, in that year the Spaniards, led by Cortés, arrived. Can you guess what happened next? That's right. The Aztecs only went and assumed that the explorer Cortés was Quetzalcoatl himself and offered him his kingdom back, no questions asked. They also made him a nice cup of hot chocolate and gave him a comfy throne to sit on.

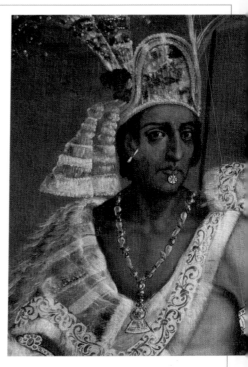

RIGHT *Montezuma—king of the Aztecs or king of chocolate drinkers? He certainly knew how to make the most of the cacao bean.*

Montezuma explained to Cortés that he personally drank some fifty cups of hot chocolate a day to give him the strength to service his vast collection of wives—around one hundred it is said—which gives us the first clue to chocolate's reputation as an aphrodisiac. Could it be that Cortés gave the game away by not taking to the miracle drink of the gods and was therefore recognized as an impostor? Whatever the reason, Cortés was caught, but it was too late for the Aztec Emperor, and he was thrown into chains. The rest is history. The Aztecs are no more, but their legacy is still very much with us.

PLANTING CHOCOLATE

Once Cortés realized the potential of cacao, he began to set up plantations all round the Caribbean, and before long there were further cacao plantations being set up in Mexico, Peru, Ecuador, Haiti, and Venezuela. The Spanish came looking for El Dorado, the city of gold, and they found chocolate instead. But the cacao bean might as well have been gold.

It appeared that the seeds could be traded for anything—one hundred bought you a slave, ten a night with a prostitute, and four a decent meal. The Jesuits called them "blessed money" and said they would free you from avarice because they couldn't be hoarded, as they rotted too easily if stored for long.

The first chocolate-processing plant was set up in Spain in 1580. The Spanish tried very hard to keep it a secret, but the information leaked out somehow, and the other European countries began to set up their own processing plants in Java and Sumatra, the Philippines, Samoa, New Guinea, and Africa.

CHEMICAL PROPERTIES

Pretty weird stuff, chocolate. It is a combination of an awful lot of chemicals, including several amino acids such as tryptophan, tyrosine, and phenylalanine, which are all well known for their ability to enhance feelings of well-being.

Chocolate also contains several natural stimulants, including caffeine (of course), but also theobromine and theophylline. These work as subtle but very effective energy pick-me-ups. You can also add to this list several calming chemicals, including valeric acid and glutamic acid. No wonder we crave chocolate and no wonder it is such a satisfying, mellow, energy-releasing, mood-lifting, and enhancing food.

RIGHT *Even eating chocolate on your own can give you a thrill. Remember to savor the taste of really good quality chocolate, and let it melt on your tongue.*

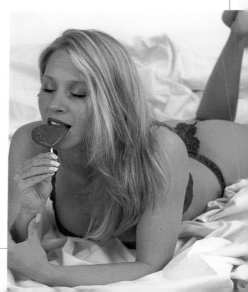

But what about the sex stuff? Well, chocolate also contains a plant substance called phytosteral that mimics human sex hormones. When women's hormone levels are low, for example when they have PMS, the craving for chocolate has been shown to be stronger and the effect of the phytosteral tends to be much more effective.

Chocolate contains over five hundred different flavors—over two-and-one-half times more than any other food known to humankind, which is why it should be tasted slowly, savored subtly, and enjoyed often. If you give them time, your tastebuds can identify all those five hundred flavors

LEFT *Luscious lips biting into a melting chocolate—the stuff dreams are made of? Make this a reality for you and your partner.*

individually, even if you can't. Wolfing down chocolate may satisfy you on a chemical level—you're getting your fix—but it doesn't satisfy you on an emotional and sensual level. For that, you really need to let your tastebuds have time to sort out all of those flavors so you can really experience them to perfection.

RIGHT *Biting into the smooth, dark surface of a single chocolate can be exciting and sensual, especially if someone is watching you.*

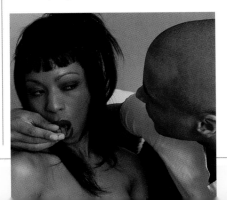

HOW CHOCOLATE HAS CHANGED

Until the eighteenth century, chocolate was known simply as "cacao."
It hadn't yet acquired its botanical name of Theobroma cacao.

It was the Swedish botanist Linnaeus who first named it so, taking *theo* ("gods") and *broma* ("drink") from the Latin and *cacao* from the original Indian—to create *Theobroma cacao*, "the drink of the gods."

You wouldn't recognize the drink the Aztecs knew as chocolate. Today's hot chocolate simply bears no resemblance to it in looks or in taste. The Aztec's chocolate was a dark and

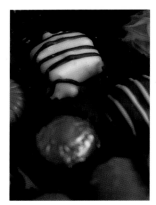

ABOVE AND RIGHT *There are so many chocolates, choosing your favorite takes time…*

grimy brew with pools of fat floating on the top—cacao butter. They used maize to soak up this fat and drank a curious sort of dark porridge with a strong bitter taste that they augmented with aniseed and chilies. But they did insist—as we do today—that chocolate should always be frothy when consumed. They poured it from a great height or stirred it with wooden paddles.

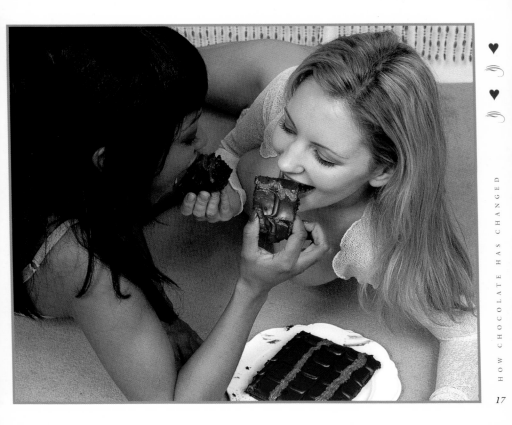

It was the Spanish sweet tooth that helped create the chocolate that we know and love today. The early processing plants stopped using chilies as a flavoring and started including delicious ingredients such as vanilla and annatto and the spice cinnamon. The chocolate was processed into large blocks—not the bars that we like today, but as a convenient and easy-to-transport base for the drinking chocolate.

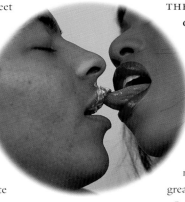

ABOVE *The lips and tongue have plenty of sensitive nerve endings—why not exploit this fact?*

Once chocolate was being processed in Spain, it didn't take the Spanish long to discover that adding sugar to the chocolate certainly improved the flavor.

THE FIRST REAL COCOA POWDER

Technically, cacao is the fruit of the tree, whereas chocolate is the processed article. But, the processed chocolate was still rich in cacao butter, which made it heavy and greasy. It was a Dutchman, Coenraad Van Houten, who developed a process to separate the butter from the chocolate. He refined this further to create a powder that could be mixed with hot water to create a palatable drinking chocolate—the first real cocoa powder. That was great, but there was still no eating chocolate for us chocoholics. Chocolate bars came about because the Dutch disliked waste. What were they to do with all that separated cacao butter? It was an easy next step to utilize this product by mixing it with a little ground cacao and sugar to create a paste that could then be dried out into blocks. This end product tasted good and could be molded and shaped into smaller blocks for more efficient and convenient handling.

In 1849, the first truly commercial eating chocolate appeared at a trade fair in Birmingham, UK. The bars were made by a company called Fry

ABOVE *A new meaning to the word sharing. Pass an ice-cold choc ice from mouth to mouth.*

that claims to this day to be the very first company ever to make eating chocolate as we know it. They were followed by Cadbury.

Eating chocolate was fairly expensive to begin with and was a luxury that was enjoyed only by the very rich. The next step was for the eating chocolate to be "exported" back to its home, the Americas. In 1900, the very first Hershey bars began to appear in many US stores, and chocolate shops soon sprang up in virtually every town. By World War II, chocolate bars were being given to the troops by the millions. Chocolate had arrived.

SECRET MEANINGS

Once chocolate bars had arrived, it didn't take long for confectionery manufacturers to start making chocolates in boxes to give and to share.

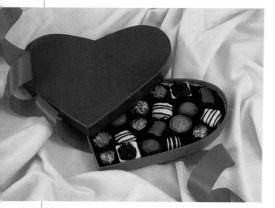

ABOVE *A beautifully presented box of chocolates can say so much to the right person.*

These early boxes of chocolates were indeed expensive but very tasty and very inventive. An early recipe book—the *Candy Cook Book* of 1917—lists over sixty fillings for chocolates, and, by that time, manufacturers were turning out over a hundred different types of chocolates.

Giving chocolates to lovers immediately became the thing to do—and quite rightly so. Giving chocolates to your loved one is a sign of love and affection. But if you are going to give chocolate, then good-quality chocolate is important. Poor-quality chocolate contains far too much sugar and can be fattening if eaten in large quantities, but good-quality chocolate is unlikely to cause weight gain as it contains far less sugar and is likely to be expensive, causing you to eat less—usually.

As well as the myth of being fattening, chocolate has spawned other myths that need dispelling. For instance, the myth that chocolate can trigger migraines in a similar way to cheese isn't true. Cheese can cause a migraine because it contains large quantities of tyramine. Chocolate, however, contains only very small quantities of tyramine and shouldn't be unfairly blamed. Likewise, chocolate is cited as a cause of acne, and this is unfair. Acne is the result of a hormonal imbalance that chocolate is more likely to correct than impair. Tooth decay has also been blamed unfairly on chocolate.

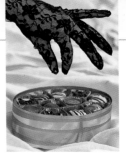

ABOVE *Pick your chocolate out with style and class, using a sexy glove as a prop.*

Chocolate melts too quickly in the mouth to cause lasting ill effects in the way that toffees and hard candies can.

So you can give chocolate freely and know that you are doing no harm, and your message shouldn't be misinterpreted. But what chocolates should you give? We mentioned expensive ones and good quality chocolate. But how do you know what is good quality? That's easy. Look at the label and check the following. The really good chocolate should have around 55–70 percent cocoa solid content, whereas cheap chocolate has only around 10 percent. The more cocoa solids, the better the chocolate. Also, be sure to check the sugar content. The higher the sugar content—and some can be around 65 percent—the poorer the quality. Very good-quality chocolate should have only around 30 percent sugar content. Reject chocolate that has vegetable fat added and also reject any chocolate with artificial flavorings.

Drinking chocolate together has definite romantic and sexual overtones, as long as it is really good-quality drinking chocolate and not a cheap cocoa substitute. Casanova drank chocolate instead of champagne. He said it was "the elixir of love."

If you want to give really sexy chocolates, the Italian chocolates known as "kisses" are very good. They are made by Perugina, and the Baci chocolates are wrapped in silver foil and contain secret romantic messages.

Dark chocolate is considered more masculine than milk chocolate and should be given to men. White chocolate is sexy and should be given to new lovers, whereas milk chocolate has more to do with love than sex. The packaging for boxes of chocolates speaks volumes. Pictures of what is inside are more important than scenes of pretty countryside. Ideally, chocolate should be wrapped in gold foil rather than cheaper silver, and the best colors to show off chocolate have always been black and red. Here's a quick list of what a lover may unconsciously be trying to say when he or she gives you chocolates:

Creams and fondants: fun and playful

Marzipan: they expect too much of you

Nougat: not to be trusted, motives dubious

Praline: too intense and obvious

Anything in a blue wrapper: it's over, they haven't the courage to tell you

Boxes with ribbons: romance not sex

RIGHT *Chocolate can be serious or it can be cheeky and playful. Experiment and have fun together.*

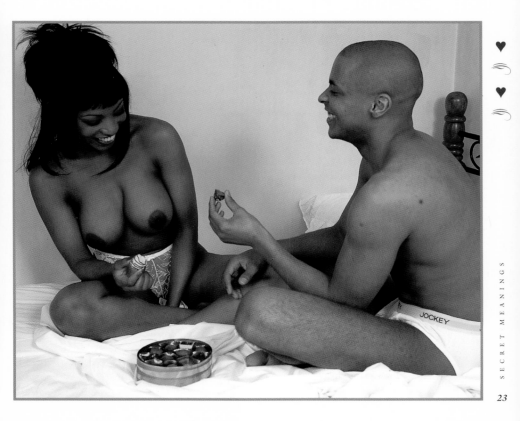

WHY CHOCOLATE IS SEXY

So why is chocolate so sexy? Well, for a whole variety of reasons. Traditionally, chocolate, especially drinking chocolate, was marketed as a health product, with wise mothers feeding it to their children in order to give them energy and stamina.

It worked for a while. But chocolate's real success has come since it has been linked to sex. And it is easy to see how and why such connections have come about. Chocolate is slinky and melting, it contains exquisite flavors, it enhances our mood, and creates a feeling of general well-being and relaxation.

UNDRESSING CHOCOLATE
We looked earlier at the content of chocolate and the fact that it contains known human sex hormone mimics. But it isn't just the

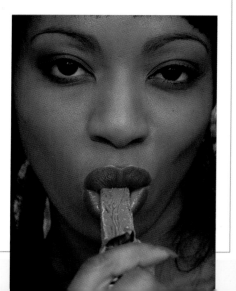

RIGHT *Undress your chocolate bar slowly and ravish it with your lips and tongue.*

chemical content that makes chocolate sexy. It is its texture, its smell, its taste, and its ability to serve as a quick fix when we're blue. It is also the way chocolate has to be unwrapped—undressed, if you like. Layers have to be peeled off before the whole naked body of the chocolate is revealed, open and ready to our gaze, waiting, anticipating our lips and tongue on its virgin surfaces. Each and every experience of chocolate is like the first experience of sex. We begin tentatively. We unwrap it slowly. We smell the delicate and heady perfume. We nibble a little, we lick, we suck, and then we greedily feast

ABOVE *Feeding chocolates to your half-dressed lover can be sexy—and lead to other things!*

on it, consuming it all in our passion and our lust. Yes, chocolate is pretty much like sex in a lot of ways.

And like sex, chocolate is versatile. If you want a quiet night at home, you can eat a box of chocolates by the fireside. If you have a taste for fancy, sexy chocolate, then there's ice-cold chocolate ice cream straight from the freezer, ready to satisfy your heat and your desire. You can have chocolate alone or share it with your lover, pushing pieces of delicious chocolate into each other's mouths in much the same way as you would indulge each other's bodies.

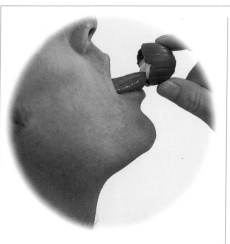

a soft, sexual, sensual, melting, tasteful experience—one to be savored, relished, and enjoyed. Only undiscerning lovers rush their chocolate, and only thoughtless chocoholics rush their sex. Sex and chocolate should both be enjoyed to the fullest. There may be time for a quickie—grabbing a bar as you rush to catch a train—but real chocolate lovers, and sex lovers of course, take their time. They seduce and titillate, flirt and woo. They don't rush, they are discerning—connoisseurs of good chocolate indeed.

RESPONDING TO PASSION

When we get sexually excited, we heat up. Our bodies become more fluid and languid. Chocolate does the same. When it heats up, it melts and becomes moist and excited. Chocolate on a cold day is hard and brittle, but chocolate in the warmth is

CHOCOLATE MAKES US WICKED

Chocolate is sexy because it is naughty and sinful, indulgent and wicked, enjoyable and satisfying to all the senses. It allows us a tiny slice of heaven on earth and is wonderful.

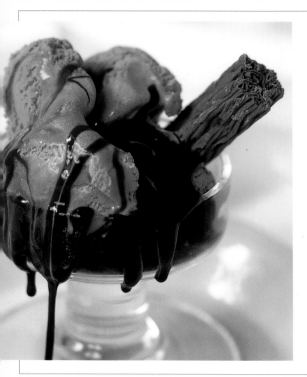

LEFT *Desserts can be very sexy.*
Go wild with the chocolate ice cream
and add oodles of chocolate sauce.

In *Madam Chocolate's Book Of Divine Indulgences,* Elaine Sherman describes chocolate as: "heavenly, mellow, sensual, deep, dark, sumptuous, gratifying, potent, dense, creamy, seductive, rich, excessive, silky, smooth, luxurious, celestial. Chocolate is downfall, happiness, pleasure, love, ecstasy, fantasy. . . . Chocolate makes us wicked, guilty, sinful, healthy, chic, happy." Stirring stuff indeed—and all of this could equally be said of sex. But can this be said of anything else? I doubt it. Sex is chocolate and chocolate is sex.

CHOCOLATE IS BETTER THAN SEX

A recent survey showed that some 20 percent of women prefer chocolate to sex, whereas 70 percent of women prefer sex to chocolate. Roughly 98 percent of men prefer sex to chocolate, and 2 percent of people polled said they liked both.

That's you, dear reader. So, is chocolate better than sex? Here's a light-hearted and fun list of thirty reasons why it is!

1. *You can always get chocolate.*

2. *You always feel like having chocolate.*

3. *Even when chocolate has gone soft, it still satisfies.*

4. *"If you love me, you'll swallow" has real meaning with chocolate.*

5. *You can safely eat chocolate while driving a car.*

6. *Chocolate will last as long as you want it to.*

7. *You can share chocolate with your mother in the room.*

8. *You can share chocolate with lots of people without it being an orgy.*

9. *You can bite the nuts in chocolate as hard as you like.*

10. *Two people of the same sex can have chocolate together without fear of being called names.*

11. *Chocolate isn't scared off by the word "commitment."*

RIGHT *Whichever partner you choose to share your chocolate with, keep it light-hearted.*

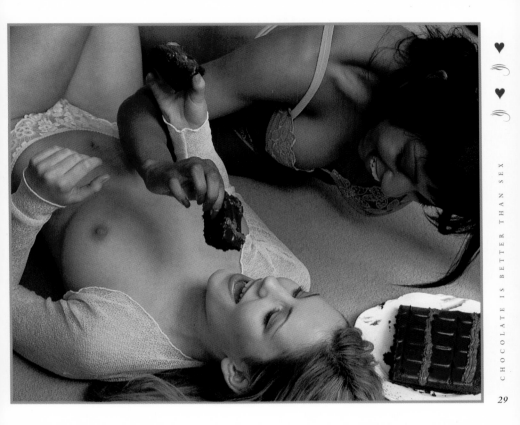

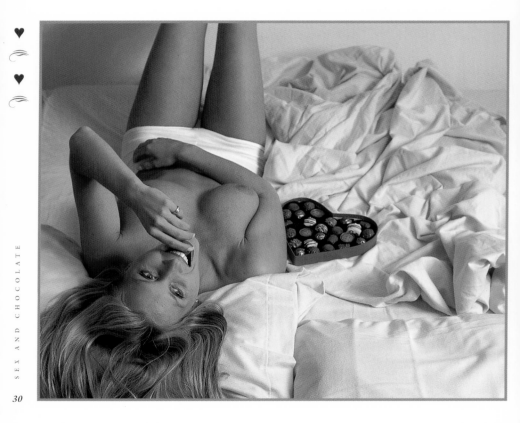

LEFT *Eat your chosen chocolates alone in bed and really make a night of it.*

12. *You can have chocolate on top of your desk at work without upsetting the boss.*

13. *It's not adulterous if you decide to switch brands.*

14. *Strangers won't slap your face if you ask them for chocolate or offer them chocolate.*

15. *You don't get hairs in your mouth when you eat chocolate.*

16. *Chocolate doesn't make you gag when you swallow.*

17. *You don't have to choose whether to spit or swallow with chocolate.*

18. *You don't ever have to fake it with chocolate.*

19. *You can eat chocolate in public.*

20. *You don't have to practice safe chocolate.*

21. *You can't get pregnant with chocolate.*

22. *Good chocolate is easy to get.*

23. *You can have chocolate at any time of the month.*

24. *You can have as many different types of chocolate as you like without people saying you're "easy."*

25. *You are never too young for chocolate.*

26. *You are never too old for chocolate.*

27. *Any chocolate is better than no chocolate; chocolate is always good.*

28. *Having chocolate late at night doesn't wake the neighbors.*

29. *Size doesn't matter with chocolate.*

30. *It's okay to go straight to sleep after having chocolate.*

All wise advice for chocoholics!

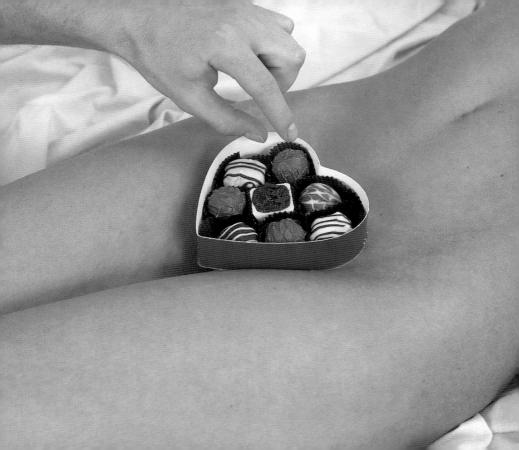

CHOCOLATE ROMANCE

*Romance is important for any loving couple, whether they are
embarking on a new relationship or are well-established in a
long-term one. Everyone needs to be romanced, wooed,
and made to feel special, and the sensual powers of chocolate can
help in this area. This isn't about jumping on your lover, covered
head to toe in chocolate ice cream, it is about taking the time to
introduce chocolate into your lovemaking and making it very
gentle, special, and right. Remember, in this instance, take it
slowly and you'll both be rewarded.*

ROMANTIC SEX AND CHOCOLATE

*To really get into the mood for romantic chocolate, we have to know
and understand the different types of chocolate and how they are best
prepared and eaten.*

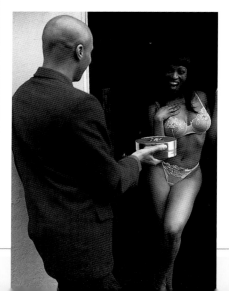

Offering your lover a bar of chocolate that is manufactured in bulk for the mass market isn't very romantic. What we need are the very best chocolates, the chocolates of the connoisseur, the champagne of chocolates. We have to pay attention to the type of chocolate as well as the wrappings, the country of origin, the fillings, and the way that they are made.

Hand-made chocolates are obviously more expensive, and they exude romance

LEFT *A man bringing chocolates to his lover might be pleasantly surprised when she opens the door!*

and thoughtfulness. And the best hand-made chocolates are wrapped exquisitely and are a beautiful and romantic accompaniment to any sexual encounter.

DIFFERENT TYPES OF CHOCOLATE

Milk chocolate is rarely regarded as proper chocolate by true chocoholics. It contains too little cacao butter—as low as 20 percent in some cheap brands, although there are some good and expensive ones with around 40 percent cacao butter—and real chocolate should have at least 60 percent.

Plain chocolate is also known as dark or bittersweet chocolate and contains a very high cacao butter content. Ideally, for really romantic chocolate you should seek out the chocolate with 70–80 percent cacao butter and a low sugar content. You and your lover want to taste the real chocolate and not some sugary candy that does nothing for your libido. Plain chocolate should also contain extract of real vanilla and not some artificial flavoring.

White chocolate may contain a high percentage of cacao butter, but it is not a real chocolate in any sense. It is sold mainly for its sweetness, as it usually has around a 50 percent sugar content. No true chocoholic would eat it, but, enjoy it as much as you can if you really like it.

Now that you know your chocolate, you should also know how to taste it. Begin first with the smell. Is it rich and not too sweet? It should be crisp and snap well when you break it. It should look smooth and clear with no indication of a "bloom," a cloudy residue on the surface of the chocolate, which is the result of too much humidity or heat during storage. Good chocolate should melt immediately in the mouth if it has not already begun to do so in your hand. Poor-quality chocolate doesn't melt so easily, despite what the ads may tell you. But it is the taste that is all-important. Good chocolate should be rich and creamy with just a hint of sweetness, not too much. It should almost zing on the tongue and be slightly bitter, causing

ABOVE *Snuggle up in the winter months and drink hot chocolate by an open fire. In your underwear, of course.*

an orgasmic explosion of flavors in your mouth when you suck on it.

SETTING THE SCENE

If you want romantic sex and chocolate, then you have to know about romance. You have to know what makes your lover's heart soar and flutter like a bird. This isn't necessarily the same as what makes their

juices flow. Romance is intimate and close rather than naughty and explicit. Romance is a whispered "I love you" and holding hands in the dark. Choosing chocolates for romance should be along the same lines—the subtle, the delicate, the restrained, and the sophisticated. A half-pound slab of milk chocolate isn't romantic. A box of delicately wrapped black and white mint cream assortments is. A bar of chocolate shared on a train late at night might be romantic. A cup of hot chocolate shared in front of an open fire by candlelight is definitely romantic.

Nakedness and romance can go hand in hand, but a little discreet covering can be even more romantic. Sharing chocolates while lying in bed is romantic, as is feeding chocolates to each other tenderly, lovingly, gently while you make tender, loving, and gentle love. There is, of course, a time and a place for hot, steamy sex and chocolate where you both just want to tear each other's clothes off, smear chocolate over each other, and lick it all off passionately. But there is also a time and place for gentle, lingering sex where you both take the time and the trouble to satisfy each other in a very warm and loving way. This is lovemaking with chocolates—chocolate romance.

BELOW *Gentle kisses that share the taste of sweet chocolate are infinitely romantic.*

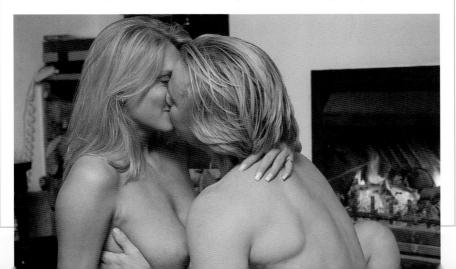

ELEGANT CHOCOLATE

The more expensive the chocolate the better it usually is—and the more elegant.
Elegant chocolate is finely wrapped, exquisitely presented, and delicate to the taste.
Some of the finest restaurants know all about chocolate desserts.

Elegant chocolate desserts are generally small to avoid any suggestion that you might gain weight. They are delicately flavored so as not to overpower other flavors in a meal, and they are made of the finest chocolate ingredients so you feel almost honored to be allowed to eat them. Elegant chocolate is not "death by chocolate." Elegant chocolate is not eating as much chocolate as you can until you feel sick. Elegant chocolate is less rather than more,

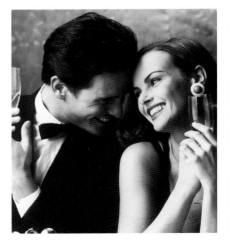

RIGHT *An elegant dinner party, where you can flirt delicately with your lover, is a great titillation.*

delicate rather than overblown, subtle rather than obvious, refined rather than coarse. Elegant chocolate is for adults who know the rules of seduction and flirtation. A tiny amount of chocolate licked from a spoon in the right way says much, much more than pigging out on a ton of cheap candy.

CHOCOLATE FOR GROWN-UPS

When we were young, we ate chocolate pudding covered in chocolate sauce. We ate so much we couldn't move. We were school children who didn't understand refinement or discernment. Now that we are adults, we know the difference. We can enjoy elegant chocolate by fine-tuning our senses and indulging ourselves in only the very, very best. A little hot mocha rum soufflé or a chocolate amaretto peach is better than

RIGHT *Dessert may be something quite different from a wafer-thin slice of chocolate cake!*

chocolate mud pudding. This doesn't mean these things are wrong—just out of place when we want elegant sex and chocolate. Being elegant and dressing for dinner are more sexy when we don't over-eat and know there will be undressing for dessert.

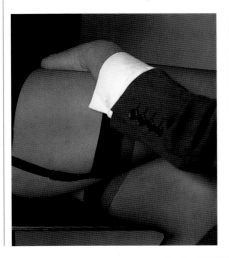

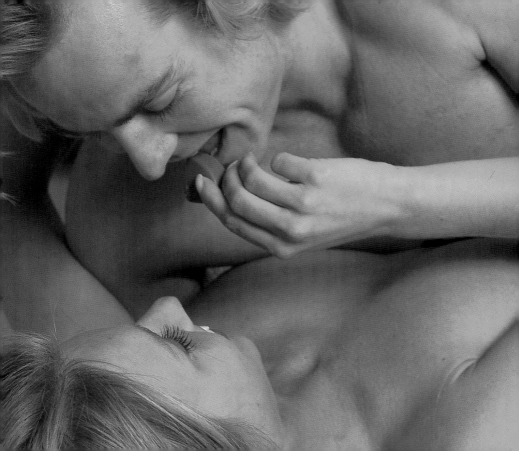

SEDUCTIVE
CHOCOLATE

For the whole of the last century, men knew that when they turned up at a lady's place for an evening date they ought to bring flowers and chocolates if they wanted to woo the woman properly. These days it's just as likely that the woman will turn up bearing gifts, and she will make her feelings known and do the seducing. Fair play. Whoever seduces whom, whoever has the job of bringing the chocolates, it doesn't matter. What matters is that you both feel free to enjoy yourselves, to seduce and flatter, coax out of clothes, lure into bed, turn each other on, and generally have a good time.

CHOCOLATE AS A SEX AID

It doesn't matter who brings the chocolates. It doesn't matter who suggests to whom that they go to bed. It doesn't even matter if the chocolates never get eaten.

What matters is respect and mutual pleasure. What matters is that you take the time and trouble to bring a gift. Bringing the gift of chocolates says many things. It says you went to some effort and that you put some thought into your seduction.

These things are good. They imply thought, respect, and care. Good sex is about not rushing. Good sex is about taking your time and enjoying each other's company, just as much as it is about what parts go where. Presented well, a box of chocolates is as much of a sex aid as anything you're likely to buy in a sex shop, and is generally much more subtle and erotic.

WHAT TO DO WITH THE CHOCOLATE
You may decide to have a little chocolate sauce on hand to paint in the shape of a heart on your lover's belly or a pair of lips for you to kiss and lick off. A little sauce poured into the navel and licked out is very sexy. Obviously, if you are going for seductive chocolate and sex, rather than out and out hard-core sex, you need to use only a little and very discreetly. Maybe sharing a bite of chocolate as you kiss is more seductive than painting each other from head to foot!

RIGHT *Passing chocolate from mouth to mouth while making love is a chocoholic's dream.*

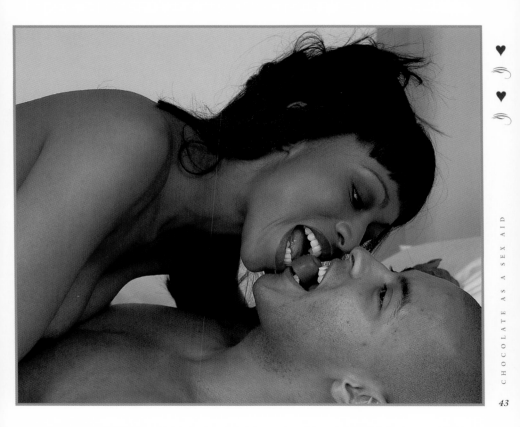

43

CHOCOLATE EROTICA

Once you've been romantic and seductive, there might be time
to be erotic with chocolate—and lots of other food of course.

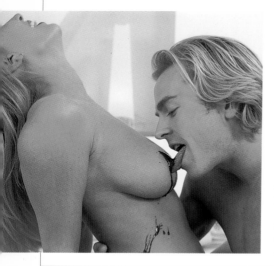

When we are first dating, we are quite restrained about what we do and what we want to do. But once we have established sufficient trust and openness, then we can feel free to discuss and discover our real sexual natures. Some of us like to continue with "normal" lovemaking and don't want to experiment—but a lot of us do.

We want our lovemaking to be playful and fun. The idea of covering our lover's nipples in chocolate sauce and licking it off appeals to our erotic side. There is some-

LEFT *Covering a nipple with chocolate sauce is a good way to get a chocolate fix and please your lover.*

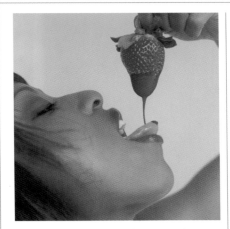

ABOVE *Strawberries are a good
erotic fruit to dip in warm chocolate
and either eat or play with.*

with our desires and our preferences. Just so long as we have sex—and chocolate—in an atmosphere of respect and trust, there is nothing wrong with playing around with our and our lover's passions.

MAKING IT VERY NAUGHTY

Some foods are very suggestive by themselves. Who hasn't looked at their lover eating a banana and thought, "If you were a lady, you'd eat that sideways?" Who hasn't been turned on by their lover biting into an ice-cold strawberry while the juice trickles down their lips in the heat of a summer's day? Sales of chocolate phalluses aren't based on their novelty value alone—they combine our two greatest and most basic needs, food and sex. Watching a woman biting into a chocolate phallus fills men with anticipation and slight fear. It is a primordial and erotic act that turns us on. And

thing very erotic and sexy about using our lover's body as a giant plate to eat food off of, smear food into and on, and, of course, lick it all clean afterward. We want to have fun and laugh a lot, as well as experiment

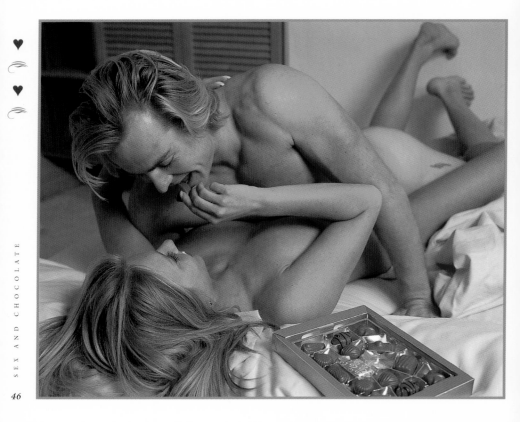

the woman herself enjoys the experience just as much because it satisfies a deeper, darker desire that only she can know.

PARADISE AND ECSTASY

Liquid cream poured over our lover's erogenous zones is erotic. But much more so when it is chocolate sauce. This is the forbidden heaven. We can use our tongues to lick up all that delicious, sweet, gooey sauce and bring them to orgasm at the same time. This is the chocoholic's paradise, the sexual experimenter's ecstasy. Imagine the effect of dipping a banana in chocolate sauce and then rubbing it lightly over your lover's nipples while they squirm with pleasure. You can then lick the chocolate off and suck

LEFT *Pushing gooey chocolates into your lover's mouth as he orgasms can raise the temperature even more.*

hard as you rub the banana in other places—and then eat it. Imagine dipping your fingers into warm, runny chocolate sauce and then pushing your fingers into your lover's mouth while they suck hard on your fingers and caress you elsewhere at the same time.

Imagine biting into a chocolate liqueur and letting your lover suck all that delicious juice out. Imagine a hot-fudge sundae eaten while you are both naked outside on a warm day as you suggestively run your fingers over your body, pausing only to dip your fingers into all that delicious chocolate and smearing it over yourself as your lover does the same. Or how about a cold white-chocolate raspberry-ripple ice cream? Make your chocolate erotic, make it sexy, make it gooey and deliciously, meltingly decadent. Most of all, make it fun.

CHOCOLATE FANTASIA

There are limits. I know this is hard to believe, but there are some things
we simply can't ask our lover to do—or shouldn't want to anyway.

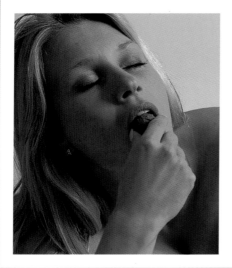

Some of these fantasies may simply be impractical to achieve—but we can still dream. Some of them may well involve chocolate. And for some of us chocoholics, all of them may involve chocolate.

TAKING THE LID OFF

Once we start exploring our fantasies, we take the lid off the private passions we have that we should probably keep to ourselves. While we might fantasize about having sex—and chocolate—with lots of different

LEFT *An orgasm and a chocolate, please—what more could a girl want or need?*

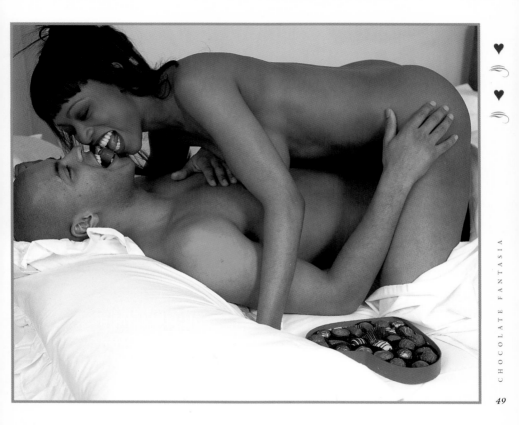

people or someone famous, our lover may not appreciate that this is only a fantasy that we have absolutely no intention of putting into practice in real life. Private fantasies are just that—private. Now that we've made that clear, we can take the lid off. Let's start with the usual "lots of people" fantasy. It's OK—we all indulge in this one from time to time. We often start off with just a couple of people of the opposite sex making love to us while we eat really exquisitely delicious chocolate—or maybe people of the same sex. That's the beauty of a fantasy, we can imagine anything we want—even if, in real life, we might not go down that road. Once we've incorporated a

LEFT *Pour melted chocolate over your lover's bare breasts and try and catch the drops with your mouth and tongue.*

couple of people into our fantasy, it's not a big step to offer an open invitation to lots. Imagine wallowing in a bath of warm chocolate sauce with fifteen or twenty or even fifty people, all squishing chocolate all over their bodies in the most erotic and sexy way. Imagine all those people using their fingers and lips and tongues on each other while someone serves fantastic chocolate cake lovingly prepared by a team of naked cooks.

RUNNING WILD

Maybe this is all too much for you. Perhaps your fantasies are quieter—just you and your lover making love while you gorge yourself on chocolate. But this needn't be a fantasy, this is one you could easily make happen. Let your imagination run wild through the chocolate avenues of your mind. Let everyone be naked. Let them all be chocolate.

Imagine being tied naked to a table while a team of erotically clad chefs cover you in chocolate sauce and layers of chocolate sponge cake and cream. Imagine you are the dessert. Imagine all of the guests filing in to look at you in wonder. Imagine them all kneeling to eat at the temple of your body. What pleasures could you imagine all those tongues and lips and fingers giving to your body? And imagine inserting a chocolate bar into a vagina—or having one inserted. This sort of thing should be worth at least a few minutes of your fantasy time—and let your partner in on the idea as well. You never know, he might enjoy the idea of eating his most favorite chocolate bar out of the most intimate place in his partner's body! Just try it and see...

COOKING WITH CHOCOLATE

Now this isn't a conventional cookbook, so don't expect too many recipes. What we are interested in are a few really good recipes for you and your partner to enjoy cooking together in the kitchen—always a good place to combine sex and chocolate.

That old kitchen table wasn't just made for your plates, you know—oh no, it can take a lot more weight than that. Try out the following recipes at your leisure, but consider cooking them in the nude.

CHOCOLATE MOUSSE

It's easy to go out and buy chocolate mousse—but where's the fun in that? You can make chocolate mousse together—and then try out the chocolate mousse games that follow. Mousse makes a delightful mess as well as tasting very good. You will need:

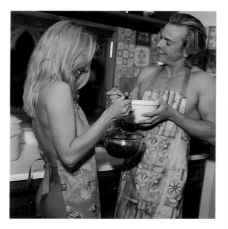

6 oz semisweet chocolate, broken into pieces

2 tablespoons strong black coffee

4 eggs, separated

1 tablespoon rum

½ pint fresh heavy cream

TO DECORATE

1 tablespoon grated chocolate

Put the chocolate pieces and the coffee into a heat-proof bowl in a pan of hot water and gently heat until the chocolate melts, stirring occasionally. Take the bowl out of the hot water and leave to cool for a couple of minutes. Beat the egg yolks and gradually stir into the chocolate mixture. Stir in the rum. Beat the egg whites in a clean mixing bowl until stiff—you may find it quicker to use an electric whisk. Carefully fold into the chocolate mixture until the ingredients are thoroughly combined. Chill in the refrigerator for a couple of hours until you are hungry enough to eat it!

CHOCOLATE CHIP CHEESECAKE

This is a truly wicked recipe that will make a delightful snack break. You will need:

4 eggs, separated

24 oz cream cheese, broken into pieces

½ cup brown sugar

2 tablespoons vanilla extract

1 cup sour cream

½ cup butter, melted

1 lb crumbled graham crackers

1 lb chocolate chips

Preheat the oven to 325°F. Prepare the batter by placing the egg yolks in a food processor for five seconds, then add the cream cheese and beat until smooth. Add the brown sugar and vanilla and process for several minutes, or until the batter is very smooth. Add the sour cream, then beat the egg whites and fold into the cheese mixture. Leave this mixture to the side while you prepare the crust. Soften the butter and mix in with the crumbled graham crackers. Mix until they form a ball when squeezed in your hand. Pat the crust into the sides and bottom of a circular baking pan about 9 inches in diameter. Spread a generous layer of chocolate chips on the bottom of the pan, and then pour the batter into the pan. Add another generous layer of chocolate chips to the top of the cake. Place the filled pan in the preheated oven. Baking time will vary from about 30 minutes to two hours. The longer you cook it, the fluffier it gets. If the cake wobbles when shaken, it is done.

CHOCOLATE PANCAKES

This is a marvelous recipe for filling hungry lovers who need refreshments to energize them after lots of lovely physical exercise. They are also quick and very easy to cook. You'll need:

½ cup margarine
½ cup cocoa powder
2 cups flour
¼ teaspoon salt
4 eggs
1½ cups sugar
2 teaspoons vanilla extract
½ cup whipped cream

Melt the margarine and mix with the cocoa. In a small bowl, mix the flour and salt. In a large mixing bowl, beat the eggs, then add the sugar and vanilla and beat well. Add the flour and margarine mixture and blend well. Heat a small skillet to a medium heat. Take small spoonfuls of the mixture and cook the pancakes for 1½ minutes on one side, ½ minute on the other then turn over again and remove after a few seconds.

*RIGHT **Aprons are only needed to cover the bare necessities as chocolate reigns supreme in the kitchen.***

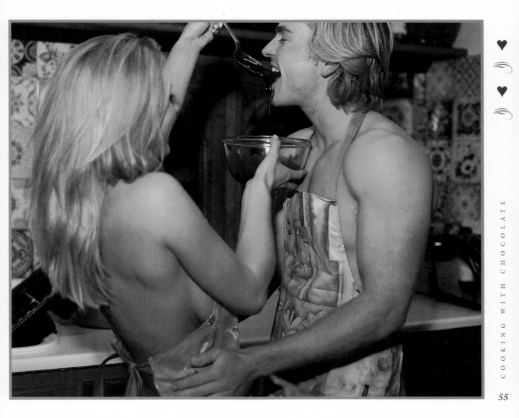

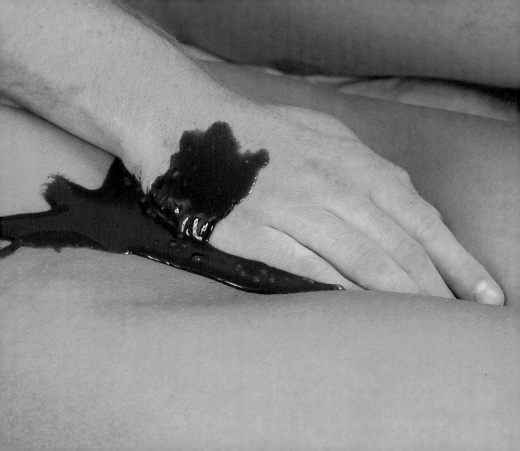

CHOCOLATE
FOREPLAY

*There is nothing better than fooling around with chocolate to get
you both in the mood. Being messy with chocolate helps break
down inhibitions—how can you take yourself seriously if you are
smeared from head to foot in delicious sticky, gooey chocolate?*

Even just eating a little chocolate together can be considered foreplay if it's done in the right way.

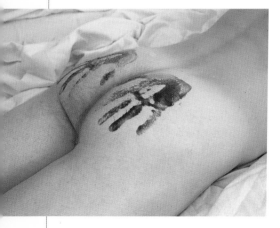

ABOVE *Make your mark on your partner's body, and leave two chocolate handprints for posterity.*

You have to be a bit imaginative—and suggestive. Unwrap that bar slowly and deliberately. Make it clear that what you are unwrapping isn't just a bar of candy but your partner's body as well.

For us chocoholics, all foreplay begins with a little chocolate—and then a lot of sex, with a lot of chocolate. Lovers know that chocolates imply desire, and that eating chocolate together is a courtship ritual, a prelude to making love.

If you want to fool around and smear yourself with chocolate, that's fine. But perhaps something a little more discreet will get your juices flowing, so save the

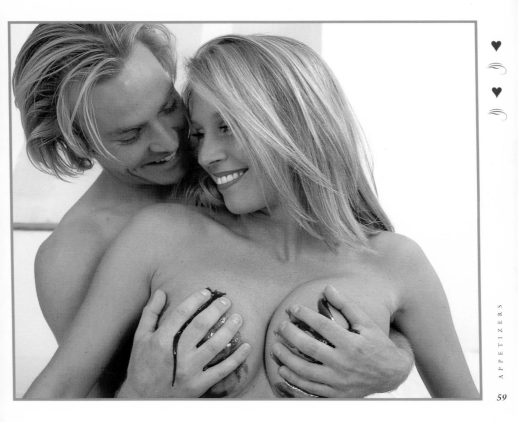

chocolate until you are both truly excited. To begin with, you could undress each other while passing chocolates from mouth to mouth. Or give a chocolate as a reward for each item of clothing your partner is prepared to take off.

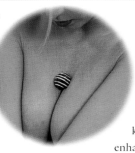

LEFT *A sumptuous chocolate cries out to be balanced on warm, sexy cleavage.*

A BALANCED DIET OF CHOCOLATE

Once you are both undressed, or as undressed as you want to be (and a little sexy underwear may be even more exciting than complete nudity), then you can balance chocolates on each other's erogenous zones and eat them off without using your fingers. A chocolate balanced precariously on a nipple needs a lot of delicacy while being licked. Some bits of the body take chocolate better than others. The navel is a wonderful place for a dark and delicious chocolate, and so are the armpits and the crook of the knee. Any woman's cleavage is enhanced by a delicately balanced chocolate nestling between her breasts, ready to be seductively taken up by a lover's lips. And once you are both naked and in the mood, then the real chocolate fun can begin. Remember all that wonderful chocolate mousse you made? Well, now is the time to use it...

The one great thing about chocolate mousse—apart from its taste—is how delightfully messy and creamy it is, so you might need to do a little preparation beforehand. Get a large plastic sheet as well as a huge roll of plastic wrap. Choose a warm room with as little carpeting as possible in case any mousse gets loose. Cover the floor with the plastic sheet and yourselves with the mousse. Wrap each other up in as much plastic wrap as you like. As the wrap gets pulled tighter, the mousse spreads wonderfully, outlining body shapes with chocolate and curves with cream.

If you want to go all out, you may need to tear holes in the plastic wrap to get access to each other's bodies, and you'll need the plastic sheet to roll around on. You might, however, just like to fool around a little and enjoy the feel of the mousse on your skin. You can lick off as much as you like—this surely is the very best foreplay imaginable.

When you've finished, you can make your way to the bathroom and wash each other clean—paying special attention to certain parts, of course.

If you don't like the plastic wrap, you can just eat mousse off each other's bodies, using your fingers and tongue—definitely no spoons allowed!

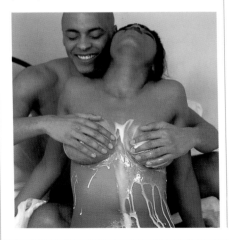

LEFT *White chocolate rubbed over bare skin warms up and covers the body sensually—and stickily!*

ORAL CHOCOLATE

Chocolate is a delight on the tastebuds, so why not combine it with the most sensual sexual experience of all? Using your tongue on your lover's body, and using chocolate too, can make for an orgasmic taste explosion.

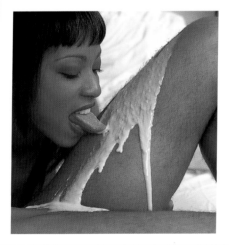

TASTE AND TEXTURE

Is oral sex foreplay or real sex? Does it really matter? Once you have made yourselves truly messy with chocolate—or just eaten enough to get you in the mood—you can indulge in a total taste fest and bring the taste of your partner's body into play. Our tongues are incredibly sensitive, and oral sex is a way of allowing all that sensitivity to be brought into play. Oral sex allows us to really experience our partner's unique taste and texture. Combine this with the delights of chocolate, and you might just discover the ultimate sexual experience.

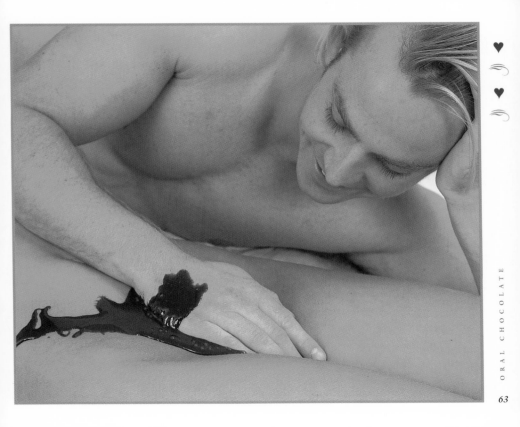

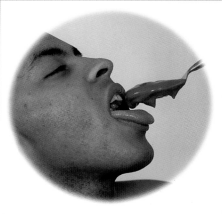

goes for oral sex. In fact, in a lot of countries, oral sex is still against the law. In reality, though, like chocolate, oral sex is pleasurable, enjoyable, sensual, passionate, and respectful. Pleasuring your partner with your tongue and lips and fingers is all part of an adult sexual relationship and can be enjoyed as part of normal and intimate lovemaking as well as an essential part of foreplay and seduction.

CHOCOLATE SAUCE

Oral sex gives us lots of excuses to pour chocolate sauce lovingly over our partner's erogenous zones in order to lick it all off—and make them reach new heights of dizzy orgasmic bliss as well. Make sure you get a chocolate sauce that isn't too rich or too sweet. The same is true of chocolate sauce as with anything else in life—the more you pay, the better you get. Invest in a really

NAUGHTY AND SINFUL

We mentioned earlier that chocolate has over five hundred different flavors—more than two and half times as many as any other food—so imagine what it is like when you add to that the delicious flavor of your partner's body. Chocolate has always been somehow "naughty" or "sinful." The same good-quality chocolate sauce and use it sparingly. A little dribbled over your erogenous zones is much more erotic than loads poured everywhere. Use a little and you can concentrate more on making things really exciting for your partner rather than clearing up the mess you've made.

HOT AND COLD

Chocolate goes particularly well with changes of temperature. You have the delicious warmth of hot chocolate and the delightfully erotic sharpness of cold chocolate ice cream. It can be fun to alternate between these two extremes of temperature to surprise your lover. Take a mouthful of warm hot chocolate and then pleasure your partner's parts. Then swallow it and take a mouthful of delicious cold chocolate ice cream and hear them scream with pleasure. The secret is never to let them know which they are going to get—if they expect heat, give them cold; if they expect cold, give them heat. Keep them guessing. Keep them squirming. Keep them coming.

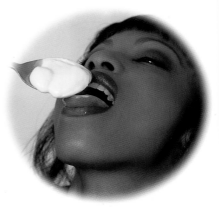

ABOVE *Cold chocolate sauces can be dropped into the mouth and other warm parts of the body.*

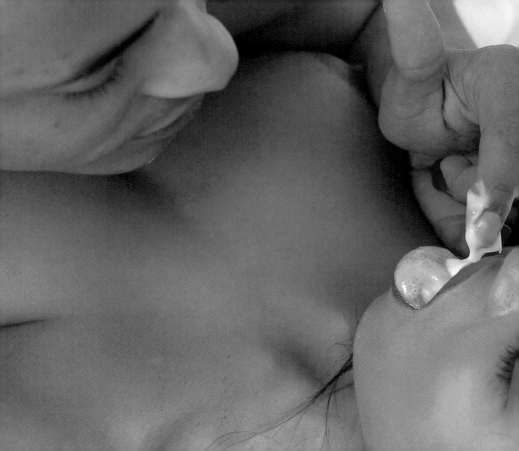

CHOCOLATE SEX

Now we get down—if you'll pardon the expression—to the real business of sex and chocolate. This is what you've all been waiting for. This is the reason why you bought this book. And why not? Combining our two great loves—sex and chocolate—can't be a bad thing, can it? The only difference is that you'll get a laugh at a dinner party if you suddenly announce you're a chocoholic, but imagine the response you'd get if you announced you are a sexaholic. The place would be in an uproar. Your lover would disown you. Your host would throw you out. Your friends would shun you. But we are all sexaholics, we just don't all admit to it. We all love to be loved, to be touched, to be caressed, to be wooed, flattered, seduced, and, well, basically, be ravished.

HAVING REGULAR CHOCOLATE

*We all need to have sex regularly. Without it we get grumpy
and lose our vitality. Look at any honeymooning couple and
you will see energy, radiance, and vivacity.*

Look at any estranged couple and you will see aging, tiredness, and a dour expression. That's what no sex does for you, and it's the same with chocolate. Chocolate eaters are happy and content people who know what's good in life, and chocolate-less people are missing one of the great things in life! They are melancholy and repressed, sad and lonely. Chocoholics are upbeat and lively. We know where our heaven is. We have found our El Dorado. And when we have great sex as well as great chocolate, then we are truly in Nirvana. If you let your imagination run away with you and experience no-holds-barred great sex, you will wake each morning feeling refreshed, invigorated, and renewed.

And what would you do if there were no rules? Well, there aren't. You could camp outdoors and cook marshmallows in front of an open fire, dip them in hot chocolate sauce, and eat them before rolling yourselves onto a blanket and making love while the fire illuminates your naked bodies in flickering shadows that are truly erotic.

RIGHT *Marshmallows dipped in
chocolate are an age-old favorite
and can be sexy as well.*

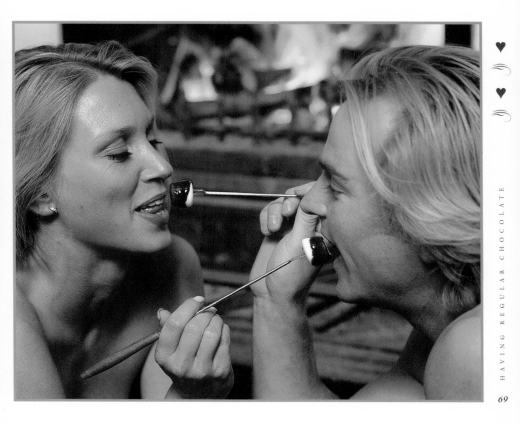

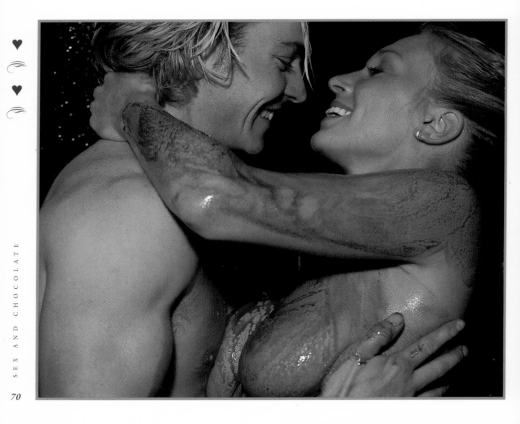

AT HOME FOR CHOCOLATE

What if you don't like the mosquito bites or being watched by park rangers? Easy. Have great chocolate at home. You'll need to set aside an entire evening. Sex and chocolate are not for quickie lovers or a one-night stand. You need to set aside time to appreciate the great gift Quetzalcoatl gave us when the serpent god brought chocolate to earth for the benefit of all humankind.

If you like slow and lingeringly delightful sex, then make love, and as you orgasm, have your lover gently push delicious, squishy chocolate into your mouth—the runnier the better so it is already melting into your mouth as you come, making your tastebuds go wild with

LEFT *There's never a better excuse to shower with each other than when you're covered in chocolate!*

sensation. Or, as you orgasm, suck chocolate from your lover's fingers in a delicious riot of passion. How about making your partner orgasm while they eat a chocolate ice cream? You have to make them come before they finish the ice cream, or you have to pay a forfeit. They might like to lose anyway! All that delicious melting ice cream may well drip with the heat of the moment and have to be licked from every orifice. If you are really up for it, the man could cover his penis in ice cream and insert it—if he can maintain an erection with all that cold—and see how his lover reacts. Could be fun. Could be interesting. Could be orgasmic.

THE CHOCOLATE TABLE

If the man stands behind his partner with her back to him, and she bends over, he can enter her from behind, while using her back as a table to rest that delicious box of exquisite chocolates on. He could offer her a chocolate, one for every thrust, or every ten thrusts, or whatever you both decide. He can also rub the chocolates against her nipples and breasts, so they melt with the heat of her body, before pushing them into her mouth. Or you can change places. The man can stand in front of her and bend forward. She can then use his back as the table and feed him chocolates as she reaches around to masturbate him. Or she can sit astride him and use his chest as a table.

For a male chocoholic there is no experience more pleasurable than watching your lover sitting above you, breasts swinging wildly, as she pumps her hips up and down on your erect chocolate-hood and feeds you chocolate truffles at the same time. You will orgasm in a wild, delightful climax of sex and chocolate that may just be heaven on earth.

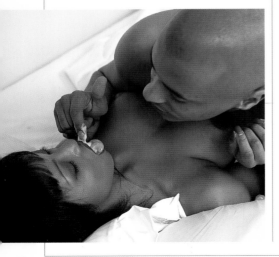

LEFT *Delicately dribble white chocolate sauce into your partner's mouth while you make love.*

RIGHT *Or, feed your lover chocolates as you both orgasm in an explosion of sex and chocolate.*

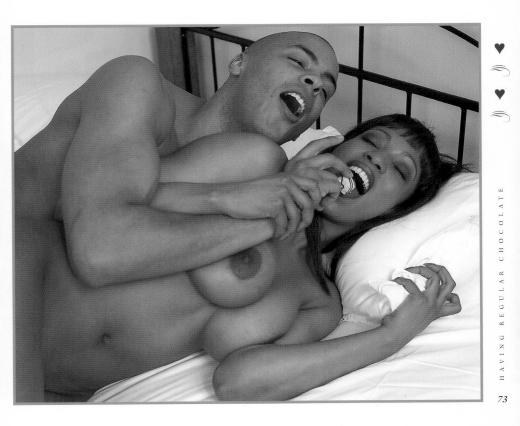

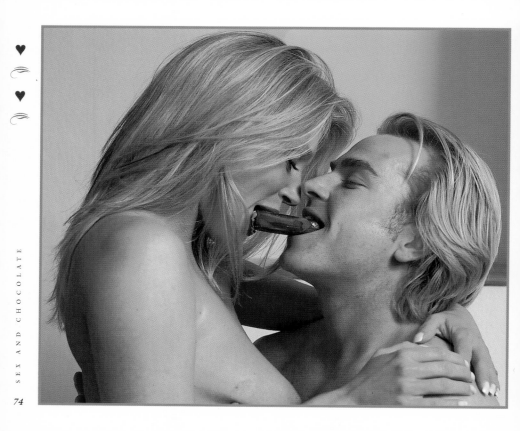

THE MISSING LINKS

There are sixty-four different love-making positions in the Indian *Kama Sutra*. Not one of them involves chocolate. In the *French Chef's Guide to Chocolate Cooking* there are over seventy recipes for chocolate eatables, but not one of them involves sex. Both books are fabulous, but both are missing an essential ingredient. We don't have space here to list the sixty-four positions or the seventy recipes, but you can do your own research and cleverly combine the two to find your own unique sex and chocolate positions and recipes. You can do it standing up, lying down, sitting astride each other, from behind, from in front, face-to-face, back-to-back, kneeling, straddling, scissoring, energetically or gently, with silk

LEFT *Sharing a chocolate ice cream can be as messy as you make it. Remember this and exploit it.*

or with ropes, with clothes or naked, in bed or outdoors, fast or slow, raunchy or romantic. The choice is yours. You can do it on a bed of profiteroles or while eating delicate slices of chocolate marzipan, with sorbet or pecan torte, with chocolate-mint ice cream, chocolate sundaes, chocolate-cinnamon doughnuts, or hot-chocolate butterscotch sauce. You choose.

The possibilities really are endless. Once you have had sex and chocolate, you may find it difficult to return to plain old sex or plain old chocolate. Once you've opened Pandora's chocolate box of lovemaking, you won't be able to close the lid ever again. Be warned. This combination is addictive and extremely pleasurable. You may never again be able to just have sex or just have chocolate. Never again will you be able to go into a store and buy a bar of chocolate without getting aroused.

DEATH BY SEX AND CHOCOLATE

*Sometimes, just sometimes, it is fun to totally overdo
both the chocolate and the sex—death by sex and chocolate.*

Make the biggest, fanciest, gooiest chocolate cake imaginable and take it to bed with you. Eat as much as you can, smear it over each other, writhe around naked, and see how far you can get on a full stomach—and a chocolate high.

Eating chocolates while making love can easily become addictive. Occasionally, it is great fun to eat too much and totally overindulge. It is a pretty wild experience to be pleasured both sexually and orally (pardon the pun) while seeing how much cake you can eat before you orgasm or exhaust yourself by laughing too much.

Alternatively, you can take the largest and most decadent box of high-class chocolates to bed with you and try to eat as many as you can during foreplay and while you make love. Balance chocolates on your lover's erogenous zones while you caress the rest of his or her body. Try to eat the same chocolate while you both bring each other to orgasm. See how many you can eat before you both feel tired and sleepy. Chocolate is very versatile, so use your very well-developed imaginations to the full and really make the most of it.

RIGHT *Sleeping off the chocolate
and sex fest is sometimes necessary.*

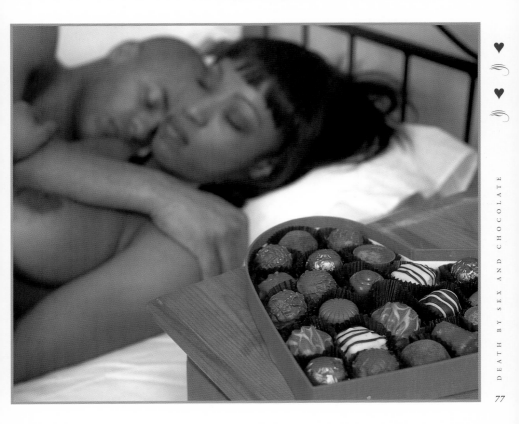

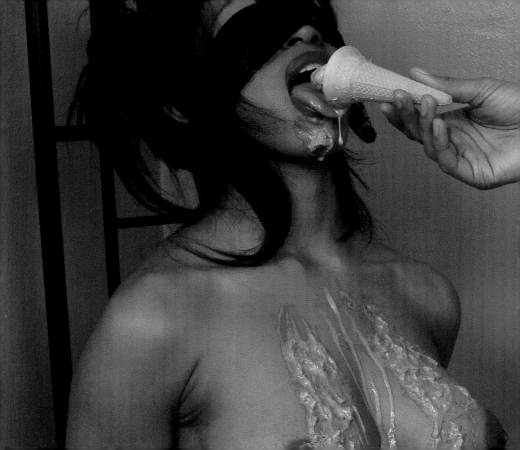

CHOCOLATE GAMES

If chocolate is for children and sex is for adults how are we ever going to have fun? The answer is easy; play sexy chocolate games and enjoy a second childhood while having raunchy, fun, and wonderful sex. What follows are some seriously silly sex and chocolate games to be played in the privacy of your own bedroom—or wherever sounds like fun. Games for you to make a mess and have some good fun together. Be prepared for some drips and don't blame us if your best satin sheets get covered in chocolate—you've been warned. And do try to get hold of really good quality chocolate even if you are just going to smear it over each other.

CHOCOLATE FUN

*As a part of sexual foreplay, toe sucking wasn't particularly
in vogue until fairly recently when several celebrities have done their
utmost to make it a popular pastime.*

You obviously need good foot hygiene for this, so this game is best played after a bath. Reflexologists say that there are more nerve endings in the feet than anywhere else in the human body. True or not, the feet—and especially the toes—are very sensitive and enjoy being sucked, licked, and kissed. Having our toes sucked does seem to have a high squirm factor. It sends delicious shivers up the whole leg to the parts where there definitely are a lot of nerve endings.

Having your toes sucked means your lover cares a lot about you, enough to overcome any inhibitions about this new and novel form of sexplay. It also means you need to be trusting and relaxed. Toes are a private and intimate part of the body, and allowing your lover access to them signals a very high degree of trust and respect indeed.

For this game you could also try using a thicker chocolate sauce and painting it onto your lover's toes. Let this sauce go hard and then slip the entire chocolate toe off and eat it in front of your partner—very strange, a little weird, very erotic.

RIGHT *Soft, clean feet covered in
white chocolate sauce can be sucked on
as a lollipop for the night.*

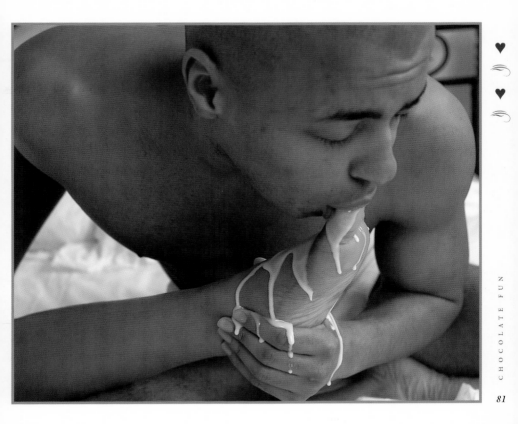

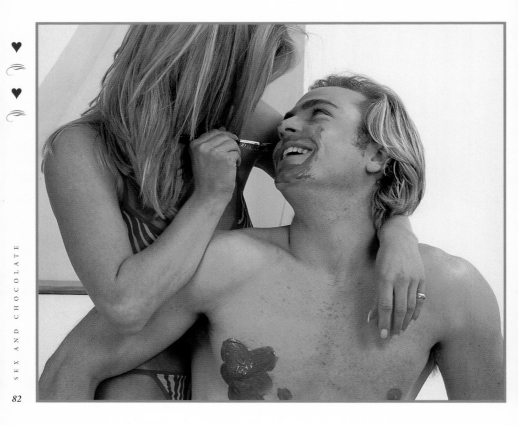

PAINTING NIPPLES

Nipples are lovely little mounds of sensual pleasure that simply cry out to be painted in chocolate that will be licked and sucked off. Make the most of your nipples and your lover's nipples. Nipples are fun. Nipples are sexy. Nipples are very sensitive. Try using very cold chocolate sauce straight from the fridge on one nipple and warmed chocolate sauce on the other. What effect does this have on your lover? Try licking one clean and sucking the other clean. You could both paint your nipples and then rub them against each other, smearing chocolate all over your breasts and chest. Warm chocolate sauce has a lovely, squishy, gooey feel to it that slides erotically across surfaces in a new and novel way.

NIPPLE MOLDS

If you use thicker chocolate sauce you can paint the nipples and wait until the sauce goes hard. Then peel off the chocolate nipple and eat it in front of your lover in as sexy a way as you can.

This kind of thing may not appeal to everyone, but try and get into the sex and chocolate spirit and do new things with your lover. Remember that this is a game and one that should be fun and silly and that you should enjoy. If your lover's nipples are particularly sensitive, then let your lover paint yours. Try painting each other's nipples while blindfolded and see what sort of a mess you can get each other into.

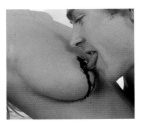

LEFT AND ABOVE *Carefully paint on chocolate face and body paint, and then lick everything off.*

CHOCOLATE HANDPRINTS

For this game, you will need a pair of dice, some thick chocolate sauce, and a small paint brush. You take turns rolling the dice, and the highest score wins each round. Odd numbers are the woman's body and even numbers are the man's body (except for the 12, see below). The higher the number the more risky a place for a handprint. Here's the all-important scoring list:

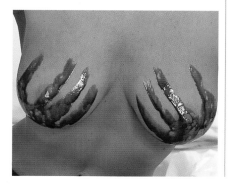

2 woman puts a chocolate handprint on man's arm; if the man threw the 2, he has to put the handprint on his own arm—get the idea?

3 woman's arm
4 man's leg
5 woman's leg
6 man's stomach
7 woman's stomach
8 man's buttocks
9 woman's buttocks
10 man's nipples
11 woman's nipples
12 man's penis/woman's vagina

Obviously the double six means real fun, but you also get to throw again. You could work out your own forfeits and dares also, but handprints will make you both laugh a lot.

LEFT AND RIGHT *You can have a lot of fun with chocolates and a pair of dice.*

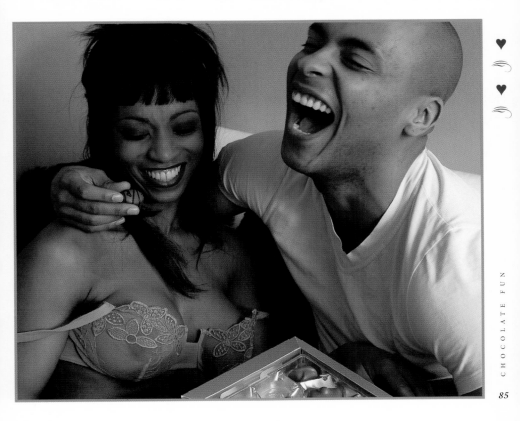

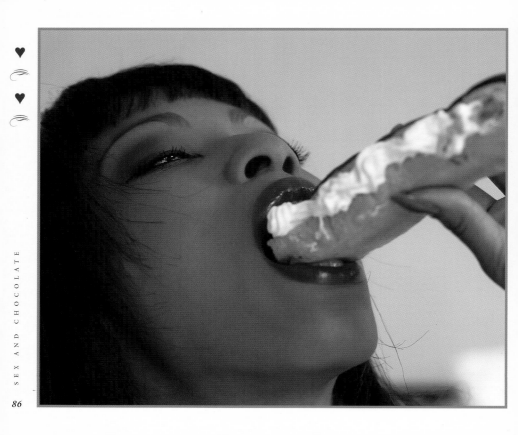

CHOCOLATE ÉCLAIR

Imagine your lover sitting opposite you completely naked—or dressed in his or her sexiest underwear—eating a chocolate éclair in the most suggestive and erotic way. What thoughts would you have? How would your juices be flowing? Well, that's the game we are going to play—orgasm by éclair.

You will need to buy some chocolate éclairs—as good quality and expensive as possible, and they should be filled with real cream. Sit opposite your lover and eat the éclair in the most lewd and suggestive way imaginable. Smear as much of the cream on yourself as you want to—or need to. Use your fingers to masturbate yourself as you eat this delicious and sexy cake. Your lover

LEFT *That's one sexy cake. Use an oozing chocolate éclair to titillate your lover and turn yourself on.*

has to sit and watch but is not allowed to touch you—or themselves. Imagine the torture and the exquisite teasing that will be felt in both mind and body.

USING THE ÉCLAIR AS A PROP

Remember you are not eating the éclair because you are hungry. Oh no, you are using the éclair as a very erotic and sexy prop, a theatrical prop to induce feelings of sexiness and eroticism. You can be as dramatic as you want to be, running your tongue up and down the sides of the éclair with just a hint of delicious cream on your tongue tip, sucking the chocolate off the top with slurping noises that will drive your lover wild, or gently nibbling on the tasty pastry as if you were nibbling on his or her body. This can be electric, and using food as an erotic aid is something we simply don't do often enough.

EROTIC CARD GAMES

In this game, we are using chocolate not so much as a sexy treat but as an aid to gambling—not just ordinary gambling, but gambling for sexual favors in a new and novel way. You will need a pack of cards and a pack of chocolate buttons. Since these are your gambling chips, divide them equally so you both start with the same amount; if you eat any you have less to gamble with.

WHAT GAMES?

You could start with strip poker—assuming you know the rules, that is—or strip blackjack naked. You can play any normal game, such as rummy or blackjack, but the person who ends up with either of the two black jacks has to remove an article of clothing. You'll need the chocolate buttons as chips to gamble with to make the game much more interesting.

WHAT FAVORS?

Once one of you has won all the other's chocolate buttons, you get to choose which sexual favor you want your partner to perform on you or for you.

You could ask them to masturbate in front of you, bring you to orgasm orally, or make love to you in your favorite position. Or you could go even further than that: you could dare them to run around the block naked, make them tie you up, blindfold you, and then cover you in chocolate sauce and lick it all off—whatever turns you on. Let your imagination run riot and your hidden desires bubble to the surface. Once you have won, you have a sexual slave who has to do whatever you want. Imagine what you could make them do.

RIGHT *A new twist on strip poker— chocolate strip poker! Think of some sexy forfeits for your willing victim.*

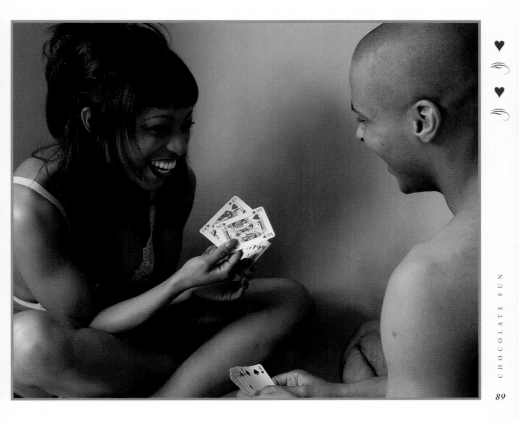

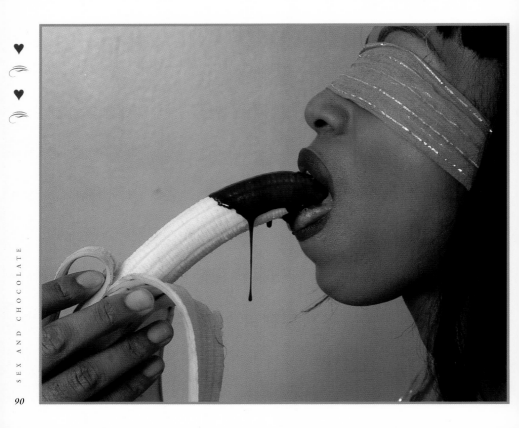

GUESSING GAMES

For this game you will need your lover, a blindfold, and a good supply of erotic fruit and food such as bananas, ice cream, yogurt, and strawberries. You will also need a large napkin and lots of chocolate sauce.

BEFORE YOU BEGIN

To start this game, you need to get your lover naked—how you do this is entirely up to you. Once naked, you must get your partner to sit in a fairly upright chair, such as a kitchen chair. Tie their hands behind their back so they can't be used. Then blindfold them and drape the napkin around their neck to keep them clean (you can dispense with this if you would prefer to make them messy). Now you are ready to begin.

LEFT *What more could you want? A banana covered in chocolate and your blindfolded partner.*

WHAT TO DO

Start off with a chocolate—the sort you get from a box—and push it gently into her mouth. She has to guess what it is. That's easy. Now try a little chocolate ice cream. Then a strawberry. Then a strawberry dipped in ice cream. Now a nipple—your own nipple, of course—dipped into the ice cream. Remind her not to bite, but only to lick. She has to guess each item put in her mouth. You can award sexual favors for a right answer and deduct sexual favors for a wrong answer. If you want your partner to win, you can make it easy. If you want her to lose, then make it difficult. Difficult is when you smear strawberry juice over a nipple, dip it in ice cream, and then layer that with some ordinary cream, topping it all of with a cherry and expect your partner to guess exactly what she is licking. And then she can do the same for you.

CHOCOLATE PAINTING

Chocolate sauce is marvelous when smeared onto a naked body and licked off. But what about some delicate painting? We can do that, too. This is more a romantic mood setter than a game where only one of you wins and the other loses. Body painting in chocolate is incredibly sexy if you do it by candlelight both very gently and delicately. You could paint a masterpiece on each other's stomachs or just paint a tiny drop on an earlobe and then lick it clean.

OTHER BODY PARTS TO PAINT

How about painting each other's lips, much as you would apply lipstick? Then you could kiss—deeply and erotically, of course—and taste the chocolate. Very sexy. You could also go all the way and use the chocolate as a complete make-up make-over. One of you could be brown chocolate and the other white as a sexy contrasting picture. You can paint one another's finger and toe nails with chocolate and lick and suck it all off. Or you could paint tribal markings on each other's faces and play in your backyard at night, dancing around a camp fire and then making love under the stars.

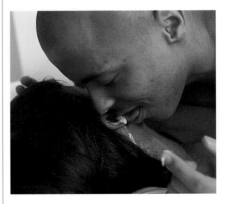

ABOVE AND RIGHT *Paint chocolate on your lover's body with your fingers or a brush.*

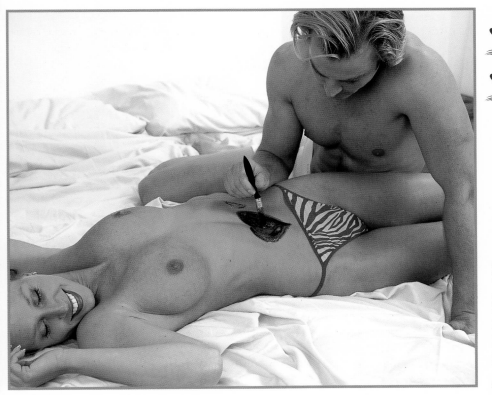

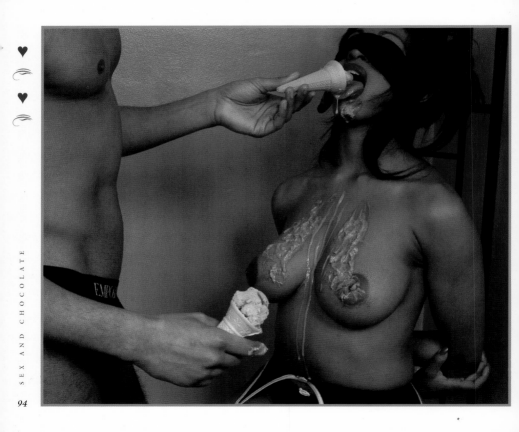

FEEDING CHOCOLATE

Sometimes just feeding each other delicious and delicate chocolates can be an incredibly sexy and romantic way to spend an evening. If you play this game, the only winning comes from being totally sexually satisfied at the end of it, and the only losing is in having to totally sexually satisfy your lover—that's not too bad, is it?

SETTING THE SCENE

Feeding each other should be erotic. Watch Albert Finney and Susannah York in the 1963 film *Tom Jones* (for which Finney won an Oscar) and you will get all the ideas you need about food (mainly apples) and sex—and in the film there is nothing explicit or raunchy, just erotic.

LEFT *Make as much mess as you can with your chocolate ice cream so you can clean it all up again...*

You don't have to dine entirely on chocolate. Try a little fruit, ice cream, and cookies. If you are spending an evening feeding each other, you will need something to drink. Champagne is better than wine, as it brings out the taste of chocolate rather than dulling it. You could, of course, drink hot chocolate, like Casanova.

Food can seem to be gender related—a banana is often seen as something a woman would eat to be sexy—but it doesn't have to. A man dipping a banana in chocolate and licking it off can be just as erotic as long as we are prepared to play around and not be too worried about sexual roles. Experiment, try new things, and be adventurous. Biting into a fresh strawberry and then kissing your lover while you let the juices run down your lips is sensual. Spooning whipped cream into each other's mouths is erotic and sexy.

CONCLUSION

In this book we have tried to give you a taste of the pleasure you can find when you combine sex and chocolate. You will find new ways of doing things yourselves, but always remember to have fun and laugh together!

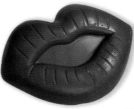

The ingredients you need are chocolate and two lovers who want to enjoy each other. There are no rules. You can do anything you want to do, as long as you both agree. There should be no pressure on either of you to do anything you don't want to do. Some lovers may not like chocolate—we assume you all like sex—in which case you may have to find an alternative, but this doesn't have to stop you from eating chocolate while making love!

Don't limit yourself to just chocolate sauce or a box of chocolates. Although these are good to start off with when you are first experimenting with chocolate and sex, there is a whole chocolatey and sensual world out there of chocolate tarts, pies and puddings, sorbets and ice creams, cookies, truffles and candies, sauces, frostings and cakes, fudges, and mousses. Have fun, have great sex, and have even greater chocolate.